MUCUSLESS DIET GUIDE BOOK

The Essential Handbook on the Mucusless Diet: Achieving a Well-Balanced Diet for a Life Free of Mucus

LARRY HERMAN

Table of Contents

Introduction

The Mucusless Diet is a dietary approach created by Arnold Ehret, a German health educator and naturopath, during the early 1900s. The main emphasis of the Mucusless Diet is on consuming items that are thought to generate mucus or produce mucus, and abstaining from such foods to enhance overall health and well-being.

Arnold Ehret's theory is based on the notion that specific foods, especially those obtained from animal sources and processed foods, play a role in the production of mucus within the body. Ehret asserts that an overabundance of mucus is regarded as a contributing factor to a wide range of health ailments, spanning from digestive troubles to long-lasting illnesses. The Mucusless Diet promotes the intake of fruits, vegetables, and unprocessed plant-based meals, which are thought to possess detoxifying and curative properties for the body.

The fundamental tenets of the Mucusless Diet encompass:

• The diet has a strong emphasis on consuming mostly plant-based foods, with a particular concentration on fruits, vegetables, nuts, seeds, and grains.

• Proponents of the Mucusless Diet frequently suggest consuming raw and unprocessed foods in order to maintain their inherent enzymes and nutritional value.

• The diet recommends avoiding the intake of mucus-forming items, including dairy products, meat, refined grains, and processed meals.

• Ehret proposed that periodic fasting or detoxification can assist in purging the body of accumulated mucus and poisons.

• **Gradual Transition:** It is recommended that followers of the Mucusless Diet transition gradually in order to give their bodies time to adapt to the changes.

It is noteworthy that although the Mucusless Diet has garnered some popularity, particularly in alternative health communities, its concepts are not universally acknowledged or endorsed by mainstream nutritionists and medical experts. Prior to adopting the Mucusless Diet, individuals should seek guidance from healthcare specialists to confirm that it is compatible with their unique health requirements and objectives.

CHAPTER ONE
The Basics of Mucus Formation

The Mucusless Diet Posits That Specific Foods Are Responsible For The Generation Of Excessive Mucus In The Body, A Condition Believed To Be Harmful To One's Well-Being. Advocates Of The Mucusless Diet Emphasize The Need Of Comprehending The Fundamentals Of Mucus Production In Order To Make Dietary Decisions That Enhance Overall Health. It Is Crucial To Acknowledge That The Viewpoints Held By Conventional Medicine May Not Necessarily Correspond With These Principles. Nevertheless, For The Purpose Of Providing Knowledge,

Below Are The Fundamental Concepts Underlying The Process Of Mucus Creation Within The Framework Of The Mucusless Diet:

• Mucus functions as an inherent defensive component in the human body, coating many organs and passageways, including the respiratory and digestive systems.

Mucus is essential for capturing and removing unwanted particles, bacteria, and irritants to prevent them from causing damage.

• **Excessive Mucus Formation:** Advocates of the Mucusless Diet claim that some foods, especially animal products and processed meals, might cause an overproduction of mucus.

• Some people claim that excessive consumption of foods that promote mucus production can lead to the buildup of mucus in the body, which may potentially cause a range of health problems.

• Foods that are thought to promote the production of mucus include dairy products (such as milk and cheese), meat, refined carbohydrates, and processed foods.

• These meals are believed to trigger the body to increase mucus production, which is assumed to contribute to the supposed adverse health effects linked to excessive mucus.

• **The Mucusless Diet Approach**: The Mucusless Diet promotes a plant-based, whole foods strategy to reduce the production of mucus.

• The focus is on ingesting fruits, vegetables, nuts, seeds, and grains that are classified as non-mucus-forming or have a lower likelihood of stimulating excessive mucus production.

5. Detoxification and Cleansing: The Mucusless Diet proposes that occasional fasting or detoxification might aid the body in eliminating accumulated mucus and pollutants.

The process of cleansing is said to promote overall health and well-being.

It is crucial to analyze these concepts with a discerning attitude and seek guidance from medical experts for tailored recommendations. Although certain individuals may derive advantages from incorporating elements of the Mucusless Diet, the scientific substantiation for the precise assertions regarding mucus production and its effects on well-being is restricted. There might be variations in how individuals respond to different dietary methods, and what may be effective for one person may not be effective for another.

Foods to Avoid

According to the Mucusless Diet philosophy developed by Arnold Ehret, certain foods are considered mucus-forming and are advised to be avoided or minimized. The idea is that these foods contribute to the production of excess mucus in the body, which is believed to be detrimental to health. Here are some of the foods that proponents of the Mucusless Diet recommend avoiding:

1. **Dairy Products:** Milk, cheese, butter, and other dairy products are considered mucus-forming and are typically discouraged on the Mucusless Diet.

2. **Meat and Animal Products:**
   Proponents of the Mucusless
   Diet suggest avoiding or
   minimizing the consumption of
   meat and animal-derived
   products, including red meat,
   poultry, fish, and eggs.

3. **Processed and Refined Foods:**
   Highly processed and refined
   foods, including white flour,
   sugar, and processed snacks,
   are often considered mucus-
   forming and are recommended
   to be avoided.

4. **Refined Grains:** White rice and
   other refined grains may be
   discouraged in favor of whole
   grains, which are believed to be
   less mucus-forming.

5. **Processed Oils:** Certain processed oils, especially those high in saturated and trans fats, may be limited in the Mucusless Diet.

6. **Caffeine and Stimulants:** Stimulants like caffeine, found in coffee and some teas, are often recommended to be reduced or eliminated.

7. **Alcohol and Tobacco:** Alcoholic beverages and tobacco products are generally discouraged in the Mucusless Diet due to their potential impact on mucus production and overall health.

8. **Artificial Additives:** Artificial additives, preservatives, and

food colorings found in processed foods may be avoided in favor of natural, whole food options.

9. **Soy Products (in some variations):** Some versions of the Mucusless Diet suggest limiting or avoiding soy products, while others may allow certain forms of minimally processed soy.

It's essential to note that the Mucusless Diet's recommendations are not universally accepted by the mainstream medical community, and scientific evidence supporting the specific claims about mucus formation is limited. Individuals considering this dietary approach should consult with healthcare professionals to ensure it aligns with their health needs and goals. As with any diet, personal preferences, cultural factors, and individual health conditions should be taken into consideration.

CHAPTER TWO
A Brief Description of Mucus-free Foods

The Term "Mucusless Foods" Pertains To A Group Of Foods That Are Thought To Be Non-Mucus-Forming Or Have A Reduced Tendency To Trigger Excessive Mucus Formation In The Body, As Outlined By The Principles Of The Mucusless Diet. The Mucusless Diet, Created By Arnold Ehret, A German Health Educator And Naturopath, Focuses On The Intake Of Plant-Based,

Whole Foods To Enhance Well-Being And Prevent The Alleged Adverse Consequences Linked To Excessive Mucus.

Here Is An Introduction To The Types Of Foods That Are Typically Considered Mucusless In The Context Of The Mucusless Diet:

• **Fruits:** Fruits Are Often Regarded As Mucusless And Are Encouraged For Their High Water Content, Natural Sugars, And Fiber. Examples Include Apples, Oranges, Berries, Melons, And Grapes.

• **Vegetables:** Non-Starchy Vegetables Are A Key Component Of The Mucusless Diet. Leafy Greens, Cruciferous Vegetables, Carrots, Cucumbers, And Bell Peppers Are Commonly Recommended.

• **Nuts And Seeds:** Nuts And Seeds, In Their Raw And Unprocessed Forms, Are Considered Mucusless Foods. Almonds, Walnuts, Flaxseeds, And Chia Seeds Are Often Included In The Diet.

• **Whole Grains:** Whole Grains, Such As Quinoa, Brown Rice, Oats, And Millet, Are Favored Over Refined Grains For Their Higher Fiber Content And Nutritional Value.

• **Legumes:** Legumes Like Lentils, Chickpeas, And Beans Are Often Included In The Mucusless Diet As Good Sources Of Plant-Based Protein And Fiber.

- **Herbs And Spices:** Many Herbs And Spices, Including Garlic, Ginger, Turmeric, And Cilantro, Are Believed To Have Cleansing And Health-Promoting Properties In The Mucusless Diet.

- **Raw Foods:** Raw, Uncooked Foods Are Emphasized To Preserve Their Natural Enzymes And Nutritional Content. Raw Salads, Smoothies, And Fresh Juices Are Commonly Included.

- **Water:** Hydration Is Considered Crucial In The Mucusless Diet, And Pure Water Is Encouraged For Its Cleansing Properties.

The Mucusless Diet Is A Distinct Dietary Philosophy With Its Own Set

Of Ideas, And Its Principles May Not Align With Current Nutritional Science. Individuals Contemplating This Dietary Plan Should Seek Advice From Healthcare Professionals To Verify It Is Compatible With Their Health Requirements And Objectives. When It Comes To Any Diet, It Is Important To Consider Balance, Variety, And Individual Preferences In Order To Have A Comprehensive And Long-Lasting Approach To Nutrition.

Transitioning to a Mucusless Diet

Transitioning to a Mucusless Diet entails gradually embracing the ideas of this dietary philosophy, which prioritizes the intake of plant-based, whole foods while eliminating or abstaining from specific mucus-forming items. Below are a series of actions and recommendations to facilitate the transition to a Mucusless Die.

• **Educate Yourself:** Learn about the principles and guidelines of the Mucusless Diet. Understand which foods are considered mucus-forming and which are regarded as mucusless.

- **Gradual Transition:** Instead of making sudden and drastic changes, consider a gradual transition. Start by incorporating more mucusless foods into your meals while reducing the intake of mucus-forming foods.

- **Emphasize Fruits and Vegetables:** Increase your intake of fruits and vegetables, especially those with high water content. Include a variety of colorful and nutrient-dense options in your daily meals.

- **Choose Whole, Unprocessed Foods:** Opt for whole grains, nuts, seeds, and legumes in their natural, unprocessed forms. Minimize the consumption of refined grains and processed foods.

- **Experiment with Raw Foods:** Explore incorporating more raw and uncooked foods into your diet. Raw salads, smoothies, and fresh juices can be delicious and nutritious additions.

- **Hydration:** Prioritize hydration by drinking plenty of water throughout the day. Water is considered a mucusless beverage and can aid in the detoxification process.

- **Mindful Eating:** Practice mindful eating by paying attention to your body's hunger and fullness cues. Listen to your body and make food choices that align with your energy and well-being.

- **Meal Planning:** Plan your meals to ensure a balanced and varied intake of mucusless foods. Experiment with different recipes and cooking methods to keep your meals interesting and satisfying.

- **Detoxification Periods:** Some proponents of the Mucusless Diet recommend short periods of fasting or detoxification to help the body eliminate accumulated mucus. Consult with healthcare professionals before attempting any detox protocols.

- **Consult with a Professional:** Before making significant changes to your diet, especially if you have underlying health conditions, consult with a healthcare professional or a registered dietitian. They can provide personalized advice based on your individual needs.

• **Listen to Your Body:** Pay attention to how your body responds to dietary changes. Everyone's body is different, so be mindful of any reactions or changes in energy levels, digestion, and overall well-being.

It's essential to approach any dietary changes with balance and consideration for your individual health needs. While the Mucusless Diet has its proponents, scientific evidence supporting its specific claims is limited. Consultation with healthcare professionals can help ensure that

your dietary choices align with your
overall health goals.

CHAPTER THREE
Meal Planning and Recipes

Meal planning on a Mucusless Diet involves selecting foods that are considered non-mucus-forming and aligning with the principles of this dietary philosophy. Here are some general guidelines and sample recipes to help you plan meals on a Mucusless Diet:

General Guidelines:

1. **Focus on Whole, Plant-Based Foods:** Prioritize fruits, vegetables, nuts, seeds, whole grains, and legumes.

2. **Incorporate Raw Foods:** Include a variety of raw foods

such as salads, fresh fruits, and smoothies.

3. **Choose Water-Rich Foods:** Opt for foods with high water content, like cucumbers, watermelon, and leafy greens.

4. **Minimize Processed Foods:** Limit or avoid processed and refined foods, including white flour, sugar, and processed oils.

5. **Experiment with Herbs and Spices:** Use herbs and spices like garlic, ginger, turmeric, and cilantro to add flavor to your meals.

6. **Stay Hydrated:** Drink plenty of water throughout the day to support detoxification.

Sample Meal Ideas:

Breakfast:

- Fruit Salad with A Variety Of Berries, Melon, And Citrus Fruits.
- Smoothie Made With Spinach, Banana, Berries, And Almond Milk.

Lunch:

- Raw Vegetable Salad with Mixed Greens, Tomatoes, Cucumbers, And Avocado.
- Quinoa Bowl with Roasted Vegetables, Chickpeas, And A Light Dressing.

Snack:

- Sliced apples with almond butter.
- Raw mixed nuts and seeds.

Dinner:

- Steamed broccoli and cauliflower with quinoa or brown rice.
- Lentil soup with plenty of vegetables.

Dessert:

- Fresh fruit sorbet made with blended frozen berries.
- Date and nut energy balls.

Mucusless Recipes:

1. **Raw Green Salad:**

- Ingredients: Mixed greens, cherry tomatoes, cucumber, avocado, lemon juice, olive oil, salt, and pepper.
- Instructions: Toss together the vegetables, drizzle with lemon juice and olive oil, season with salt and pepper.

2. **Quinoa and Vegetable Stir-Fry:**

   - Ingredients: Quinoa, broccoli, bell peppers, carrots, garlic, ginger, soy sauce.
   - Instructions: Cook quinoa. Stir-fry vegetables with garlic

and ginger, then mix with cooked quinoa and soy sauce.

3. **Mixed Berry Smoothie:**
   - Ingredients: Mixed berries (strawberries, blueberries, raspberries), banana, spinach, almond milk.
   - Instructions: Blend all ingredients until smooth.

4. **Lentil and Vegetable Soup:**
   - Ingredients: Lentils, carrots, celery, onion, garlic, vegetable broth, herbs.
   - Instructions: Sauté onions and garlic, add vegetables, lentils, and

broth. Simmer until lentils are tender.

Remember, these are just sample ideas, and you can adapt recipes based on your preferences and dietary needs. Consulting with a healthcare professional or registered dietitian can provide personalized guidance and ensure that your meal plan meets your nutritional requirements.

Detoxification and Cleansing

Transitioning to a Mucusless Diet requires progressively adopting the concepts of this dietary philosophy, which stresses the intake of plant-based, whole foods while eliminating or avoiding particular items that can produce mucus.There is no text provided.Detoxification and cleansing are commonly linked to specific dietary methods, such as the Mucusless Diet. Within the framework of the Mucusless Diet, detoxification is thought to facilitate the expulsion of accumulated mucus and toxins from the body, hence enhancing general health and well-being. It is crucial to acknowledge that although detoxification is widely discussed in alternative health practices, there is limited scientific evidence to support specific claims made about detox diets.

Within the context of the Mucusless Diet, there are several broad concepts related to detoxification and cleansing of the body through the consumption of specific foods.

Below are a series of stages and helpful suggestions for successfully shifting to a Mucusless Diet:

Periodic Fasting:

• Some proponents of the Mucusless Diet advocate for short-term fasting or periods of reduced caloric intake. This is believed to give the digestive system a break and support the body in eliminating toxins.

Raw Food Cleansing:

• The emphasis on raw, uncooked foods in the Mucusless Diet is thought to support natural detoxification processes. Raw foods are believed to retain their natural enzymes and nutrients, contributing to the cleansing of the body.

Hydration:

• Adequate hydration is considered essential for detoxification. Drinking plenty of water is believed to help flush out toxins and promote the elimination of waste products from the body.

Herbal Teas:

• Some variations of the Mucusless Diet may include the consumption of herbal teas with purported detoxifying properties. Examples include dandelion tea, ginger tea, or nettle tea.

Juice Fasting:

• Juice fasting, where individuals consume only freshly squeezed fruit and vegetable juices for a designated period, is sometimes recommended in the Mucusless Diet for its cleansing effects.

Colon Cleansing:

• Colon cleansing techniques, such as enemas or colon irrigation, are sometimes associated with detoxification practices in alternative health circles. These methods aim to remove waste and toxins from the colon.

It's crucial to approach detoxification practices with caution and under the guidance of healthcare professionals. While some people may find benefits from aspects of detoxification, extreme or prolonged fasting, as well as certain cleansing practices, can have potential risks and may not be suitable for everyone.

Before embarking on any detoxification program or making significant changes to your diet, it's advisable to consult with a healthcare professional or a registered dietitian. They can provide personalized advice based on your individual health status and needs, ensuring that any dietary changes align with your overall well-being. Additionally, keep in mind that the body has its own natural detoxification mechanisms through the liver, kidneys, and other organs.

Conclusion

Arnold Ehret established the Mucusless Diet as a nutritional philosophy that promotes the intake of entire, plant-based meals while eliminating or avoiding items that are thought to produce mucus. The fundamental concept is that an overabundance of mucus production within the body, which can be linked to specific dietary selections, might have a role in the development of diverse health problems. Although the Mucusless Diet has garnered considerable popularity, its concepts are not widely embraced by mainstream nutritionists and medical specialists.

The process of transitioning to a Mucusless Diet is progressively integrating non-mucus-forming foods, such as fruits, vegetables, nuts, seeds, and whole grains, into one's eating habits. At the same time, it requires reducing the consumption of mucus-forming foods, such as dairy, meat, and processed products. Meal planning on a Mucusless Diet can encompass a wide range of options and allow for creativity, focusing on including raw foods, maintaining proper hydration, and selecting full, unprocessed plant-based alternatives.

• The Mucusless Diet is commonly linked to detoxification and cleaning, which involve techniques including fasting, consuming raw food, and drinking herbal teas. It is crucial to exercise caution and seek the counsel of healthcare specialists when doing detoxification, as severe methods may carry possible hazards.

Prior to embracing any dietary regimen, such as the Mucusless Diet, it is imperative for consumers to seek guidance from healthcare specialists or trained dietitians to ascertain its compatibility with their unique health requirements and objectives. For a nutrition plan that is both balanced and sustainable, it is important to take into account personal preferences, cultural influences, and individual health problems. In order to substantiate the precise claims associated with the Mucusless Diet, it is essential to have scientific proof. Additionally, individuals should pay attention to how their own bodies respond to dietary changes.

THE END

www.ingramcontent.com/pod-product-compliance
Lightning Source LLC
Chambersburg PA
CBHW061314250726
48653CB00002B/930